YOGA FOR OSTEOPOROSIS

Healthy Home Exercises & Beneficial Poses You Should Do To Help You And The Ones You Should Avoid As An Osteoporosis Patient

MYLAH HARRISON

Copyright © Mylah Harrison 2023

Table Of Contents

Introduction

Yoga should be incorporated into your Osteoporosis treatment regimen. It can reduce your risk of issues, alleviate symptoms, and strengthen your bones.

Yoga may also assist to increase bone density after menopause.

Gentle yoga weight-bearing postures can help with pain treatment, strength development, and appropriate posture. It also improves agility, stability, and flexibility.

These benefits make daily activities easier, improve coordination, and reduce your risk of falling.

Learn more about the benefits of yoga for osteoporosis, poses to do, and precautions to consider.

YOGA
FOR
OSTEOPOROSIS

HEALTHY HOME EXERCISES & BENEFICIAL
POSES YOU SHOULD DO TO HELP YOU AND
THE ONES YOU SHOULD AVOID AS AN
OSTEOPOROSIS PATIENT

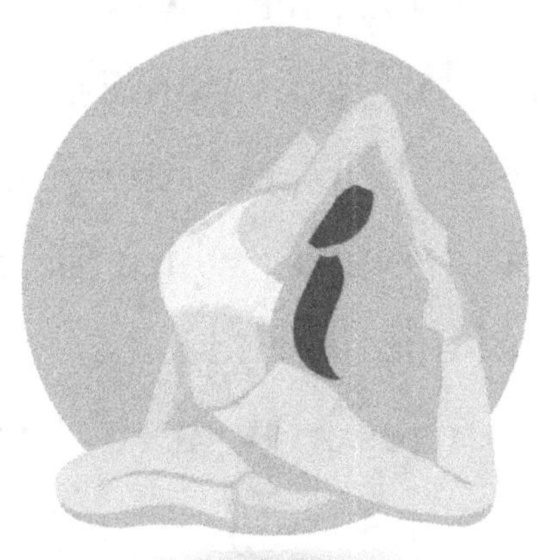

MYLAH HARRISON

Chapter 1

What You Need to Know as You Age

Yoga is an excellent way to manage symptoms of osteoporosis. A solid routine can help to strengthen your muscles and bones, which helps lower your risk of injuries and falls.

Individualities may need further to achieve good blood vitamin D situations. It's delicate getting all of that from food every day. So, you may need a vitamin D supplement to reach these pretensions.

Fit in potassium and protein:
Potassium bettered calcium
metabolism. You'll find this
mineral in fruits and vegetables,
especially bananas, potatoes(with
the skin), prunes, orange juice,
tomato juice, raisins, acorn squash,
lima sap and spinach. Get enough
protein too.

Since calcium and minerals are
bonded to interlocking protein
beaches in bones, protein is crucial
for healthy bones. In some studies,
protein has helped with bone
mending too.

Get Weight-bearing Exercise Regularly: Walking, dancing, calisthenics class, weight training "Any exertion that puts your bones to work stimulates the redoing that keeps bone strong. Start with 15 to 20 twinkles a day.

However, start by working with a physical therapist who can help you move duly to get results and stay injury-free, If you 're frail. " Cut back on caffeine and alcohol. Drinking either in excess can reduce your bone viscosity.

Quit Smoking: Tobacco use leads to significant bone loss in women and men, longer mending times after a fracture and an advanced threat for complications.

Quitting can reduce the added threat. 65 percent and the threat for other fractures by 53 percent. Side goods include skin responses at the   point of the injection, increases in blood and urine calcium, and bone pain. In high boluses, this   drug causes bone cancer called osteosarcoma in rats, but this has not been seen in people.

Chapter 2

Yoga for Osteoporosis

Yoga is a great way to control osteoporosis symptoms. By strengthening your bones and muscles, a regular exercise program can help reduce your risk of falls and injuries.

You should incorporate yoga into your treatment plan for osteoporosis.

It can lessen your chance of problems, help with symptoms, and strengthen your bones.After menopause, yoga may also help to increase bone density.

Weight-bearing postures in gentle yoga can help with pain relief, strength development, and proper posture. Additionally, it enhances agility, stability, and flexibility. These advantages facilitate daily activities, enhance coordination, and lower your chance of falling.

Find out more about the benefits of yoga for osteoporosis, as well as poses to try and safety measures to take.

Avoid emphatic styles similar to ashtanga, vinyasa, or power yoga. It's stylish to do a small quantum of yoga each day rather than many longer sessions each week.

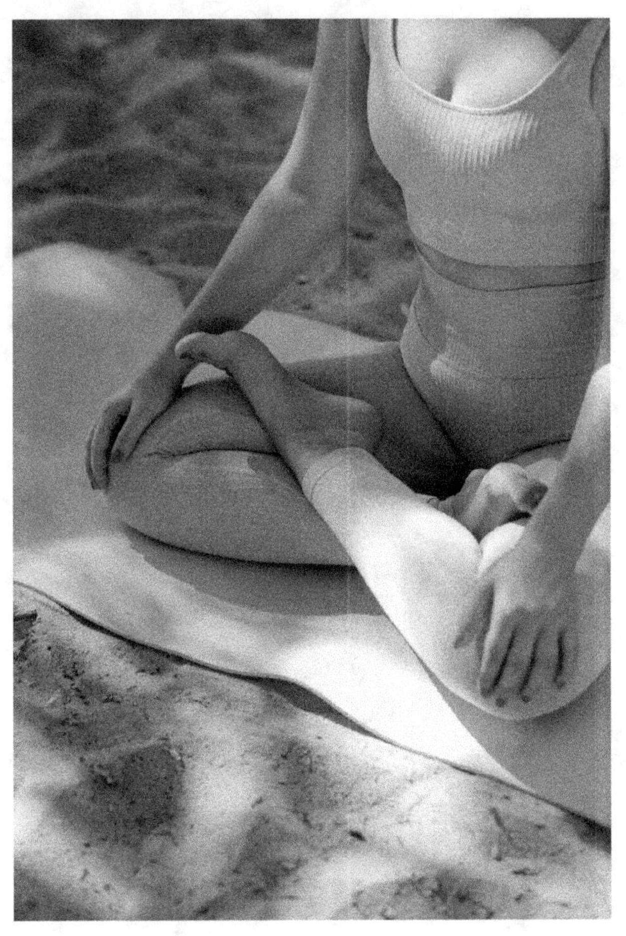

Poses To Do And Precautions To Consider

• High Plank Pose

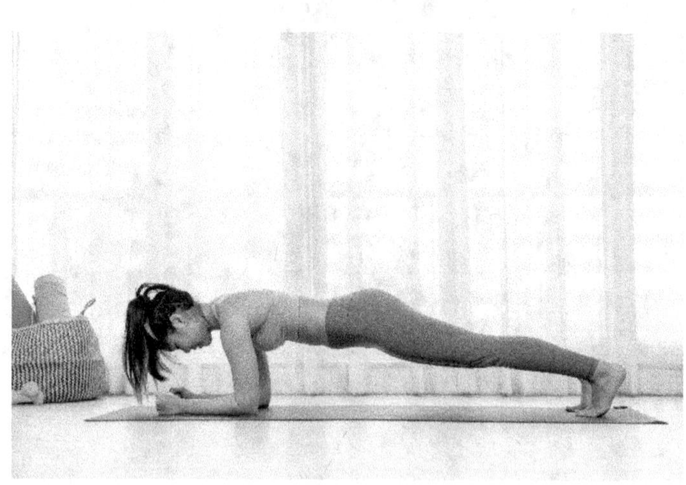

Your hamstrings, glutes, and shoulders will all get stronger with high plank pose. Additionally, it strengthens your core and back, which enhances posture and balance.

Guidelines for High Plank Pose

Take a seat at the table.
Lift your hips and straighten your knees as you push your heels back behind you.
Stretch your back and engage your arm, core, and leg muscles.

As you spread your chest wide,
bring your shoulders back.
Hold for one minute at most.
Do it one to three times.

• Downward-facing Dog

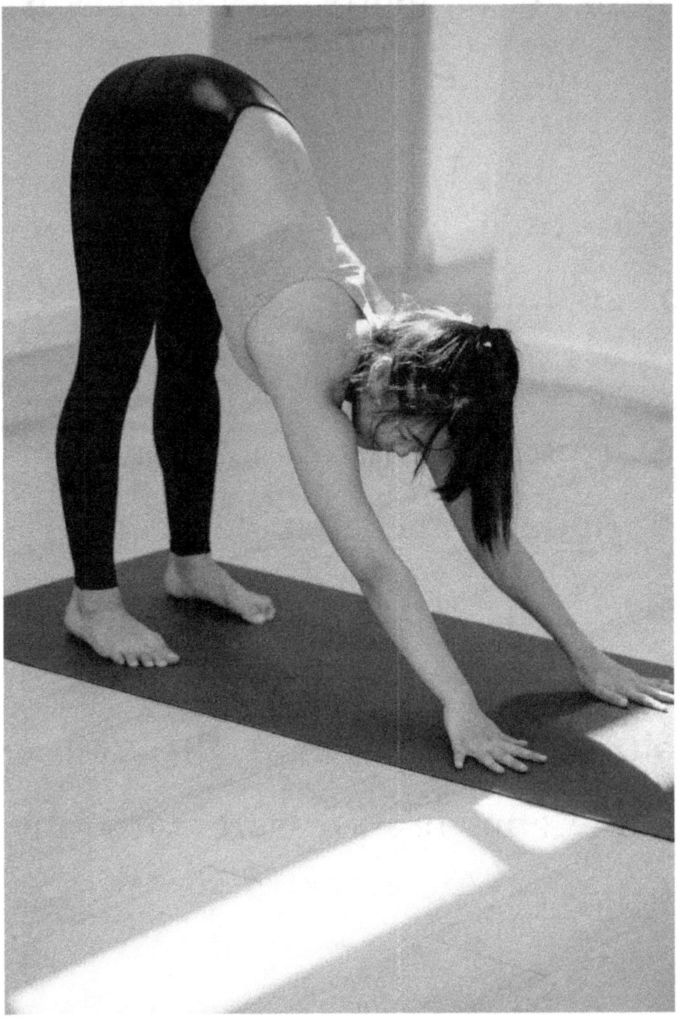

Your arms, back, and legs will all get stronger with this traditional pose. It supports proper posture and alignment of the body.

How to do the dog pose with your head down

Start in the tabletop position, heels up and toes tucked under feet.

Lengthen your spine and lift your sitting bones toward the ceiling while applying pressure with your hands.

Lengthen your spine and keep your knees slightly bent.

Either bring your chin up against your chest or align your ears with your upper arms.

Hold for one minute at most.

Do it one to three times.

• Warrior II

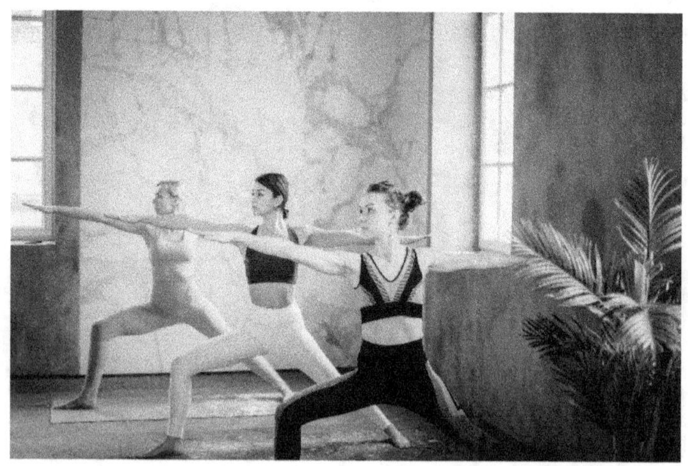

Your legs, shoulders, and chest will all get stronger in this pose. It gives your thighs, hips, and chest a mild stretch.

Performing Warrior II Pose

Step back with your left foot and point your toes slightly to the side while standing.

Turn your left hip back so that your torso is facing the side.

Raise your left arm back and your right arm forward until your palms are parallel to the ground.

Right knee should be bent slowly until it is directly above your ankle.

Keep your knee from going past your ankle.

Lengthen your spine and distribute your weight equally across both feet.

Extend your arms over your chest and extend both hands' fingertips.

Keep your eyes on your middle finger up front.

Pose for a maximum of one minute

Repeat on the opposite side.

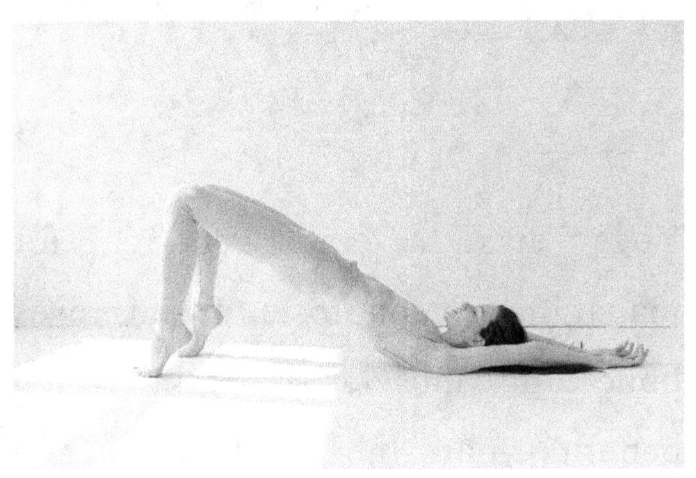

Chapter 3

Benefits Of Yoga For Osteoporosis

Yoga has several benefits for managing osteoporosis. It improves bone and muscle strength, which benefits your stability, balance, and posture. Maintaining an active lifestyle can help manage pain and lower your chance of bone fractures. Additionally, you can increase your awareness through yoga practice, which will make you more conscious of your movements.

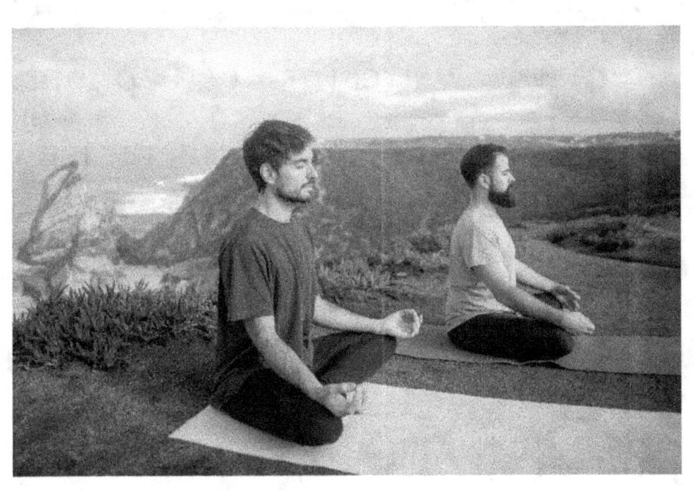

Any alternative therapy aims to cure or manage the illness without the need for prescription drugs. For osteoporosis, there are some alternative treatment options. Despite the fact that there isn't much clinical or scientific proof to support their efficacy, many users report success.

Always consult your physician before starting any alternative medication or treatment. Herbs and the medications you currently take may interact in some way. The most comprehensive treatment plan for you can be coordinated with the assistance of your physician.

Although further studies are required to fully understand the issue, certain herbs and supplements are thought to lessen or even reverse the bone loss brought on by Osteoporosis.

Red Clover

Estrogen-like compounds are thought to be present in red clover. Some alternative care providers may advise using natural estrogen to treat osteoporosis because it can help protect bone.

Red clover may help slow down bone loss, but there is no scientific proof for this claim.

Red clover's estrogen-like substances might conflict with

other prescriptions and not be appropriate for certain individuals. If you're thinking about taking red clover, make sure to talk about it with your doctor.

There are numerous potential adverse effects and drug interactions.

Tai Chi

An array of fluid and gentle body postures that flow from one to the next are used in the ancient Chinese art of tai chi.

According to research conducted by the National Center for Complementary and Integrative Health, tai chi may help older adults' immune systems and general well-being.

Additionally, it might lessen stiffness and pain in the muscles and joints and enhance muscle strength and coordination. Improved balance and physical stability can be achieved with a regular, supervised routine. It might also stop falls.

Melatonin

The pineal gland produces the hormone melatonin in your body. Melatonin has long been promoted as an all-natural anti-inflammatory and sleep aid.There is growing evidence that melatonin encourages the growth of healthy bone cells.

Melatonin is a very safe supplement that is widely available in liquid, tablet, and capsule form. However, it can make you sleepy and interfere with blood pressure, antidepressants, and beta-blockers, so consult your doctor first.

Horsetail

Horsetail is a plant with possible medicinal properties. The silicon in horsetail is believed to help with bone loss by stimulating bone regeneration. Although clinical trials to support this assertion are lacking, horsetail is still recommended by some holistic doctors as an osteoporosis treatment.

Horsetail can be taken as a tea, tincture, or herbal compress. It can interact negatively with alcohol, nicotine patches, and diuretics, and it's important to stay properly hydrated when you're using it.

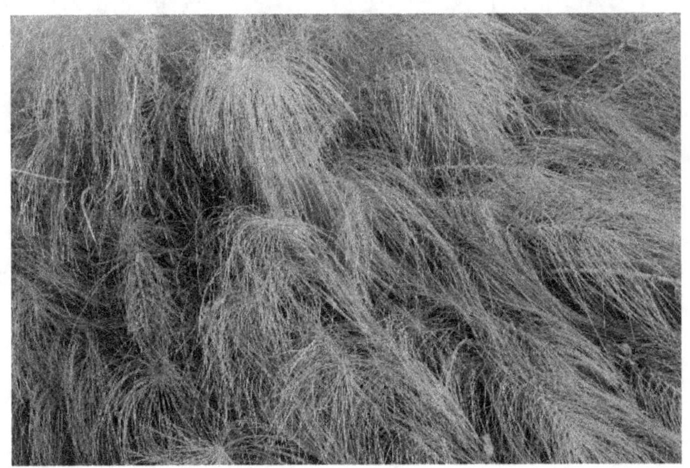

Acupuncture

Acupuncture is a therapy used in traditional Chinese medicine. The practice involves placing very thin needles in strategic points on the body.

This method is believed to stimulate various organ and body functions and promote healing. Acupuncture is often combined with herbal therapies.

While anecdotal evidence supports these as complementary osteoporosis treatments, more studies are needed before we know if they truly work.

Herbal treatments are frequently combined with acupuncture. Although there is anecdotal evidence to support these as complementary treatments for osteoporosis, further research is necessary to determine their efficacy.

Soy

The soybeans used to make products like tofu and soy milk contain isoflavones. Isoflavones are estrogen-like compounds that may help protect bones and stop bone loss.

It's generally recommended that you talk to your doctor before using soy for osteoporosis, especially if you have an increased risk of estrogen-dependent breast cancer.

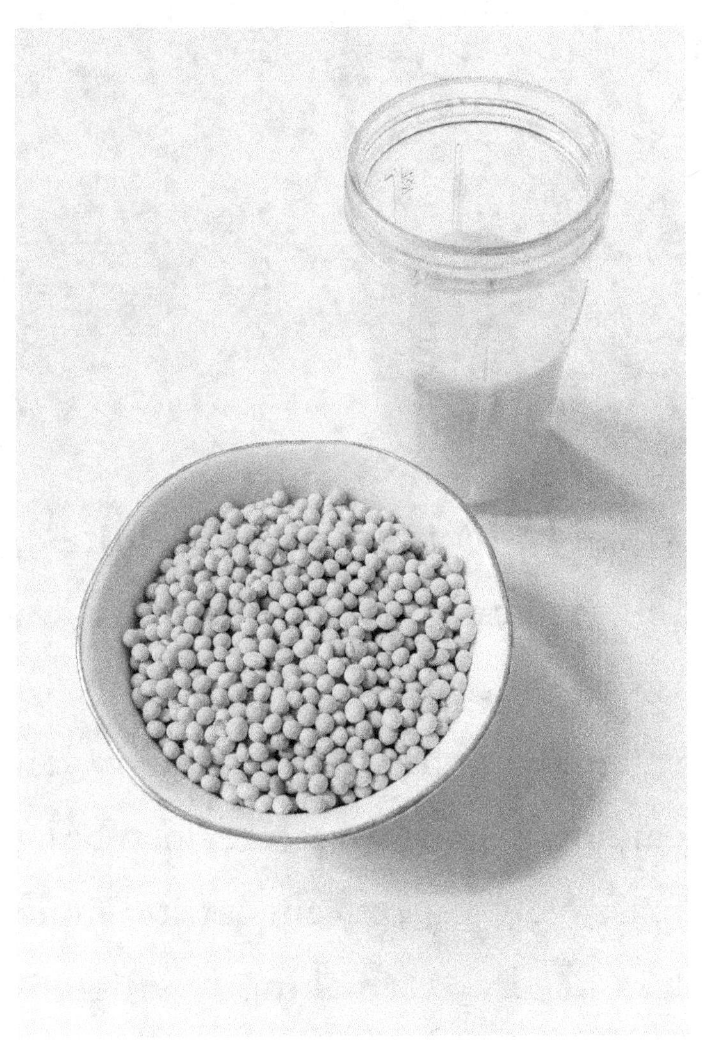

Chapter 4

Traditional Treatment Options

When osteoporosis is identified, the recommended course of action is to increase the amount of calcium in the diet. Although you cannot instantly restore lost bone mass, you can prevent further bone loss by making dietary adjustments.

It is common practice to prescribe hormone replacement medications, especially those containing estrogen. However, the side effects of all hormone therapy medications can affect other aspects of your life.

Since they prevent bone loss and lower the risk of fractures, medications in the bisphosphonate family are also frequently used as a form of treatment. Heartburn and nausea are two of this medication class's side effects.

Some opt to try alternative ways of treating their osteoporosis and halting bone loss due to the side effects of these synthetic medications. Prior to beginning any medication, always inform your physician about it.

Conclusion

In conclusion, "Yoga for Osteoporosis" presents an all-encompassing strategy for enhancing and managing bone health via the age-old discipline of yoga. In order to build bone strength, increase flexibility, and foster general well-being, we have studied a range of yoga poses, breathing exercises, and mindfulness practices throughout this book. You start down the path to maintaining bone density and developing resilience by implementing these exercises into your daily routine.

Recall that yoga promotes harmony and balance in both the body and the mind. It is not merely a physical workout. Be gentle and understanding with yourself as you proceed on your yoga path. Mindful practice and consistency are essential. Accept yoga's transformative potential as a tool for managing osteoporosis, and may this book